Essential Oils for Beginners

A proven Guide for Essential Oils and Aromatherapy for Weight Loss, Stress Relief and a better Life

Sarah Joy

information is without contract or any type of guarantee assurance.

The trademarks that are used are without any consent, and the publication of the trademark is without permission or backing by the trademark owner. All trademarks and brands within this book are for clarifying purposes only and are the owned by the owners themselves, not affiliated with this document.

Table of Contents

Introduction

You will agree with me that most people have the misconception that aromatherapy involves anything that smells good like perfumes and scented candles. However, aromatherapy refers to the use of plant essential oils normally diluted in some kind of solution for therapeutic application. These essential oils are extracted from the leaves, bark, roots, rind and flowers of plants. The oils are then mixed with another substance such as a lotion, oil or alcohol and then inhaled or sprayed in the air. You can also use essential oils in massage or bath water.

Aromatherapy originated from Europe and people have been practicing this form of alternative medicine from the early 1900s. Pioneers of aromatherapy believed that the fragrances in the oils stimulated nerves and these nerves would send impulses to the part of the brain, which controlled memories and emotions, and the result on the body would be stimulating or calming depending on the type of essential oil used. Over the years, more people have turned to the use of essential oils as an alternative medicine.

This book will help you understand the different kinds of essential oils and ways of using the different essential oils to achieve varied goals. After reading this book, you will know what essential oils to use for weight loss, better skin, pain and so much more.

What are essential oils?

Essential oils are simply volatile liquids distilled from different parts of plants such as the leaves, stems, bark, seeds, roots, fruit and flowers. An 'Oil' is considered essential in the sense that it has a distinctive essence or scent of the plant it was extracted from. A variety of factors normally determine the purity of the essential oil like geographical region, climate, the part of the plant the oil was produced from, soil condition, fertilizer, harvest methods and the distillation process.

Essential oils are not what we could consider actual oils because they do not have fatty acids. Essential oils are volatile meaning they evaporate when exposed to air, are scented, do not feel slick or oily and do not leave any oil residue.

Why it is close to impossible to find pure, therapeutic grade essential oils?

We all know that essential oils are usually available in small bottles that are quite expensive. Most of these essential oils are not usually pure since it is quite costly to produce the purest form of essential oils. Do you know that you will require hundreds or even thousands of pounds of plant material in order to produce a single pound of oil? To understand this much better, we shall evaluate the cost of one type of essential oil. A pound of Melissa essential oil for instance costs around $10000. Although this may sound outrageous, do you know that just to produce that one pound, three tons of plant materials were used. This is why a small amount of essential oil is quite expensive; hence the need to use sparingly. In any case, a little oil goes a long way.

What to look out for when buying Essential Oils

With all the craze about essential oils, there has been an increase in the number of companies selling essential oils. While there are those who may be selling pure essential oils, others are out to make some few dollars. This means that you need to be extra careful when buying essential oils. Thus, you should consider some important factors when buying essential oils to avoid being duped or using harmful substances.

All natural oil

If you see words like fragrance or aroma, like lavender aroma, you can almost be sure that it is fragrance oil rather than therapeutic oil

The Latin Botanical Name

The botanical name is important as it helps explain the origins of a particular extract. For instance, if you are looking for Lavender essential oil, you should look for Lavandula angustifolia, which is the botanical name.

Price

You need to understand that quality therapeutic essential oils are quite pricey. Thus, low priced oils are likely to be synthetic and chemical based fragrances that do not have any therapeutic benefits. Ensure that you buy your essential oils from a company that you trust and that offers in depth information about any essential oil you want to buy.

Dark glass bottles

Essential oils have to be stored in glass bottles. Thus, stay away from essential oils in plastic containers.

100% pure and undiluted

Always buy pure essential oils rather than diluted ones. While it is important to dilute an essential oil, you are better off diluting it with something that you know like jojoba oil or any other carrier oil of your choice.

Therapeutic Grade

You need to buy essential oils that are excellent quality for therapeutic applications.

How to use Essential Oils

You can use essential oils differently to enjoy their therapeutic benefits. Below are the different ways that you can use essential oils

Inhalations

When you use essential oils through inhalations, you simply use in diffusers or put the essential oil in hot water for inhalation. Inhalations are best for use if you have headaches, sinus, and respiratory problems. When using inhalations, you should inhale for short periods; roughly, three minutes since long inhalation of essential oils can cause nausea, dizziness, lethargy, headaches and vertigo.

Compresses

This involves the use of a few drops of essential oil blends dissolved in hot water and soaking a cloth in the water. Compresses are amazing for use on wounds, bruises, muscular aches, and skin problems.

Baths

If you would want to use essential oils in a bath, it is preferable to mix them first with bath salts or emulsifier like milk or sesame oil. This is because the bath salts disperse the oils safely into the water. If you do not use salts or a suitable emulsifier, the drops of essential oils will simply float on water and even get directly on the skin; something that you do not want to happen. If you were to combine the heat of the water and the essential oils, they can cause dermotoxity, especially if such oils are of a heating nature.

Aromatic baths are usually the best if you have skin problems, stress, and nervous tension, insomnia, menstrual and muscular pains.

Massage

Pure essential oils are actually 70 times more concentrated than the entire plant. Thus, if you want to do an essential oil massage, there is need for dilution with suitable carrier oil.

Facial Steam

You may use facial steam if you need to open sinuses, for skin treatment and curing headaches. What you do is simply dissolve a few drops of the essential oil in water and cover your head with a towel.

Direct palm Inhalation

When using this method, you should approach with caution. You should only use with oils that can be applied on the skin. All you need to do is apply two drops of oils to the palms, rub your palms, then inhale deeply. This is an amazing method when looking for quick and easy exposure to therapeutic uses of essential oils.

Diffusers

Diffusers are amazing for releasing essential oil scents into the air. You may need to know about the different diffusers available in the market and the benefits of one over the other.

Electric Heat Diffusers

With this diffuser, small absorbent pads are put inside a heating chamber with ventilation allowing the aromatic compounds to evaporate into the air. These diffusers are easy to use, can diffuse thicker oils and require minimal maintenance. You should however be aware that heat damages some aromatic compounds; hence, you should exercise caution.

Cool Air nebulizing diffusers

With this type of diffusers, there is a system that uses air pressure generated by a compressing unit used to vaporize the essential oils. There is usually a glass nebulizing bulb, which serves as a condenser that only allows the finest particles of essential oils to escape into the air. The greatest benefit of these diffusers is that they allow for strong diffusion; thus maximizing therapeutic benefits. These diffusers are however not suitable if you are looking to diffuse more viscous oils like ylang ylang.

Candle Diffusers

Usually, a heat resistant vessel that has water and the essential oils, and a heat resistant platform holds the vessel over a relatively small candle. This is amazing for use since it offers a light background fragrancing. The greatest problem with using candle diffusers is that they do not produce a strong concentration of oils for therapeutic benefits.

Aromatherapy And Essential Oil Therapy:
Use Of Essential Oils

Most people use aromatherapy and essential oil therapy interchangeably although they are quite different. The term "aromatherapy" is used wrongly mainly because most people think that all essential oils smell nice. On the contrary, many essential oils do not have a nice smell. Even though you can say that smell is relative, the German chamomile is an example of one of the many essential oils that do not have an appealing smell. Instead, "aromatherapy" refers to the use of essential oils through smelling and inhaling. However, you need to understand that essential oils do not need to be used through inhaling only. When talking of the other different ways of using essential oils, we use the term "essential oil therapy", since this term is more descriptive.

There are quite a number of different essential oils with each having a particular health benefit. However, before we get into the particular health benefits, let us first look at the how to use essential oils safely.

Safety Considerations When Using Essential Oils

It would be imprudent to think that just because something has immense healing power, it cannot do damage when administered incorrectly. Essential oils should be administered with care to prevent adverse effects. We will have a look at some important considerations that you need to have in mind even as you use essential oils to ensure that you use them correctly.

Age

While younger children can use essential oils, there is need for the essential oils to be further diluted owing to a young child's young skin that is likely to be highly permeable. This means that an adult cannot use the same concentration of an essential oil as a child. The dilutions (of 0.5 – to 2.5 percent) will depend on the ailment or condition being treated.

However, you should avoid essential oils containing methyl salicylate or peppermint. Oils like Birch and Wintergreen should not be used on younger children. Older people should also be careful when using essential oils as their skin may have become more sensitive over the years hence the need for further dilution using a carrier oil. We will look closely at carrier oils later on in this section.

Application

Essentials oils can be applied in various ways depending on the reason for the use. For instance, essential oils can be:

- nhaled, for example, Eucalyptus and Peppermint essential oils

- iffused, for example, Frankincense, Cinnamon bark, Oregano and Clary Sage essential oils

- ngested for example, Anise Seed, Cardamom, Fennel, Coriander seed, Peppermint, and Bergamot essential oils

- Applied on the skin, for example, Black pepper, Ginger and Chamomile essential oils

It is best to follow the instructions of use when dealing with essential oils. As far as safety is concerned, inhalation presents low risk because as the essential oils evaporate, they become diffused into the environment. When it comes to ingestion, you should not ingest anything unless explicitly instructed to do so. When it comes to skin application, ensure that you dilute the essential oils before use unless told otherwise to avoid skin irritation.

Chemical Composition

Some essential oils can cause skin irritations. These essential oils usually contain aldehydes and phenols. In order to use such essential oils, you should first dilute them using carrier oil (a vegetable oil that acts as a base for the essential oil and that dilutes the oil to keep it from irritating the skin). You can also blend them with an essential oil that can counteract the irritant effects. If you are unsure of whether or not essential oils will cause a skin irritation, ensure you do a test by applying it on only a small patch of your skin first.

Condition of the skin

You should be careful when using essential oils on skin that has been damaged or inflamed. This is because such skin is permeable to the oils and thus allows in more essential oils that would normally get into the skin. This means that the essential oils have the potential to cause greater damage especially if you are allergic to them. In order to prevent the risk of doing more damage to your skin, ensure that you only use dilutions on such skin.

Below are various dermal (skin) reactions that can come about from the use of essential oils.

Dermal irritant

This is where your skin becomes irritated after the application of the essential oil. Your skin becomes red, painful, and blotchy depending on the dilution (or lack of dilution). Essential oils made from barks are said to be more irritating than those made from plant leaves. Dermal irritants include essential oils like cinnamon, clove, lemongrass, and oregano among others.

Dermal sensitization

This condition starts subtly but over time, the application of the essential oil can cause a severe inflammatory reaction. Known dermal sensitizers include cinnamon bark, peru balsam, cassia and turpentine oil among others.

Photosensitization

This is where the application of essential oils causes your skin pigmentation to change. These 'burning' changes can be mild or severe. There are drugs like tetracycline that are known to increase photosensitivity and should be avoided when using essential oils. You should also avoid common photosensitizers such as bergamot, cumin, expressed orange, lime and lemon.

Mucous membrane irritant

Mucous membrane irritants like cinnamon, lemongrass, and peppermint should not be used in a full body bath, as they tend to dry up the mucous membrane. If you want to use such essential oils, ensure that you use a dispersant like vegetable oil first.

Dosage

Essential oils are usually diluted between one percent and five percent especially when used in blends. Three things should be considered before choosing the dosage of essential oils.

- Your sensitivity to the essential oils

- Area of application (some areas tend to be more sensitive than others)

- The essential oil used (some essential oils tend to be irritants)

It is also wise to note that if you abuse the use of essential oils, you will gradually develop sensitivity and irritation to the oils.

Despite the potential adverse effects of wrongfully administering essential oils, the benefits that come with essential oils make it worth it to learn how best to avoid the potential adverse effects.

How to use Essential Oils safely

Do not ingest

Do not ingest essential oils unless specifically told to do so on the instructions for use. Keep in mind that even though the ingredients occur naturally in the environment, the process used to extract essential oils makes them highly concentrated.

In case you ingest an essential oil not meant to be ingested, ensure that you drink milk (you can also drink soy milk or rice milk), cream, honey or yoghurt. These products will dilute the essential oil.

If your skin becomes irritated after the application of essential oils or the essential oil gets into your eyes, use vegetable oil to dilute the area and wipe off gently.

Use carrier oils

One way to dilute essential oils is by using carrier oils. These are vegetable oils that work as the base of essential oils to make them less concentrated. If you are instructed to dilute an essential oil, first pour carrier oil before adding the essential oil and then mix as per instructions (normally you can have a drop of essential oil to one teaspoon of carrier oil but this will of course depend on factors such as your sensitivity or the oil in question). There are many carrier oils, like olive oil, jojoba, coconut oil, sunflower oil, pecan oil, avocado oil, sesame oil and macadamia nut oil.

Keep essential oils from children

Children will be naturally attracted to essential oils since some of them smell nice and also because children are naturally curious. However, instead of following instructions (mostly because they cannot read at this age or comprehend the gravity of the situation), they often go ahead to drink up the whole bottle and this will of course harm them. Refer to the section for "do not ingest" to know how to handle the situation if any of this happens. Ensure to visit a doctor immediately to address the problem.

Stay away from the sun

Some essential oils are photosensitizing. They will end up giving you burns or uneven color changes if you expose your skin to the sun. Once you apply an essential oil, stay indoors, and allow the essential oil to work.

Don't use the same essential oils

Like many other medicines and healing agents, essential oils should be used interchangeably otherwise their effect will wear off or you may develop resistance or an allergic reaction to a particular essential oil. Instead of relying on just one essential oil, have several, which you can use.

Keep away from flammable substances

Essential oils can go up in flames very quickly. They are highly flammable and should be kept in a cool environment. When using essential oils, ensure that you use them in a well-ventilated room and away from flammable substances.

Always perform a skin patch test when applying essential oils on your skin

When you learn about the healing power of essential oils, you may be excited about trying them out for yourself. However, you should pause for a moment and conduct a skin patch test before continuing onto the affected area. Even if you have used other essential oils without problems, get into the habit of performing the skin patch test whenever you try out a new essential oil.

Always consult a doctor before using any essential oils

Some essential oils need to be avoided when pregnant. You should also not take some essential oils if you are epileptic or have asthma. This makes it critical to consult a health practitioner before using essential oils.

Safety precautions are there for a good reason. Don't just jump on a bandwagon because others swear on the use of a certain essential oil. As an individual, what works for another person may result in an allergic reaction when it comes to you. Always perform a skin patch test when it comes to trying out new essential oils on your skin. Once you understand how to safely administer essential oils, you can go ahead to enjoy the many benefits of essential oils.

Essential Oils And Weight Loss

Essential oils are very helpful in enabling you lose weight since they work on the part of the brain that deals with the feeling of satisfaction in addition to the breakdown and release of unwanted toxins and fat from the body. Let us look at the various ways that essential oils can work to enhance weight loss.

Use Of Essential Oils In Suppressing Appetite And Achieving Satiety

The feeling of fullness is usually regulated by a part of the hypothalamus in the brain. Our nose and olfactory nerve is also connected to this part hence our sense of smell is connected to the hypothalamus in the brain. Essential oils release scent molecules that make their way to the nasal cavity, then the mucous membrane and finally to the olfactory nerve. These molecules are then taken by the limbic lobe to the brain to allow the brain to respond to this stimulus. Since the limbic lobe is the emotional center of the brain, it sends information to the hypothalamus that has the ability to make you feel full.

Your emotional state can trigger easily the desire for food. Most restaurants and food chains use essential oils in the preparation of food to trigger cravings. We can also use the sense of smell to our favor and suppress our emotional response to food as well as our appetite. You can use various essential oils to suppress appetite and achieve satiety.

Peppermint

One of the commonly used essential oil that helps in weight loss is peppermint. Studies indicate that peppermint has an effect on the hypothalamus. Inhaling peppermint essential oil before a meal or putting a few drops in a glass of water and drinking before each meal will give you the sense of fullness.

Grapefruit

Grapefruit essential oil is useful in purging the body of retained fluids and toxins. The aroma lessens food cravings and thus is useful for weight loss. You should inhale grapefruit essential oil when cravings strike. You can also use a drop of the oil in a glass of water to stop the cravings.

Rosemary

Rosemary is well known for its effect on the brain and memory. In addition, it acts as an appetite suppressant as it stimulates the hypothalamus. Apart from enhancing satiety, rosemary is useful in detoxification. This means it helps your body get rid of excessive fluids and harmful toxins. It also improves the digestion of foods. You should have a bottle handy and sniff in the oil when hunger strikes. Sniff three times in both nostrils.

Ginger

Ginger is useful as an appetite suppressant. It also helps to improve your digestion and it increases your energy levels too. However, you need to use it with care as it tends to burn. As any other essential oil used for suppressing appetite, keep it close and sniff it when hunger strikes.

Lime

Lime essential oil is essential in fighting against cellulite, as it is rich in vitamin C. Its aroma is also useful in treating depression and boosting positive thinking. This means that not only does it help you by getting rid of cellulite, it also stops you from binge eating because it uplifts your spirits.

Basil

Basil works best as a fat burner when it is used with carrier oil. Once you have the mixture ready, you should massage the oil onto your full body. This will help emulsify your excess body fat and thus help you lose weight.

Thyme

Thyme has many useful properties that make it a powerful ally when it comes to healing. However, as a stimulant, it works to stimulate the digestive system and therefore increases metabolism. This is very useful to those who want to lose weight.

Fennel

Fennel also works to stimulate the hypothalamus in order to produce feelings of satiety. This means after inhaling it, you will feel full instead of craving food. Fennel also works to enhance positive energy. This is helpful especially to those who tend to gain weight from comfort eating as a positive outlook reduces your desire for comfort eating. You should sniff the oil several times during the day.

As you start using essential oils to control your appetite, you would need to choose three or more oils for use during the whole day. It is advisable to carry them wherever you go and use them frequently, as they are known to be effective with frequent use. When you feel that you are tempted to eat or are feeling hungry, or even before you start eating a meal, you should open the bottle and take around three whiffs in every nostril, and breathe as deeply as possible in each nostril as the other is closed. Once you are done, you should close the bottle immediately to avoid diffusing the smell. It is usually advisable to rotate the essential oils to avoid getting used to a particular one such that it no longer has any effect. You can inhale several times daily or put a few drops in water and drink depending on your needs.

Essential Oils For Achieving Calmness

Most people who gain weight are known to do so mainly because they are emotional eaters who turn to food for comfort when stressed. Bergamot essential oil is very useful when stressed since inhaling of the essential oil enables you to feel calm, and thus reduce stress levels. Therefore, you are not going to eat too much since you are not stressed. Bergamot has especially worked for me mainly because I am an emotional eater.

Essential Oils That Increase Metabolism

Increased metabolism is very important in weight loss. While there are no known essential oils that actually burn fat, essential oils can work by increasing your metabolism, which can help you to lose weight and reduce the fat deposits in your body. Grapefruit, Bergamot and Lemon essential oils are known to be very effective in increasing one's metabolism.

Although essential oils are effective in suppressing your appetite and increasing your metabolism, you still need to use them alongside a healthy diet and exercise. Do not simply expect that you will lose weight if use essential oils but still have an unhealthy diet rich in saturated fats, sugars and highly refined carbohydrates.

Essential Oils In Reducing Anxiety, Stress And Depression

Each day we face frustrations, work deadlines, and demands by both our families and the society. Many are the times that we are stressed such that stress becomes a part of our life. However, stress can influence various biological processes including management of weight, anxiety, fatigue and depression. Chronic stress can also cause hormonal adrenal and thyroid conditions.

How Essential Oils Relieve Stress

The sense of smell can greatly affect our mood mainly because the sense of smell is directly linked to the limbic system in the brain (the emotional center of the brain). What this means is that our sense of smell will not only affect our emotion but also other physical processes in the body. When we inhale essential oils, the molecules are channeled by receptors to the olfactory system. The receptors transfer the information from the molecules to the brain leading to the sense of smell. The olfactory bulb being part of the limbic system captures information through the sense of smell and records it as a memory. This is why you can smell a particular scent and immediately you have flashbacks of certain memories. Considering that the limbic system is responsible for stress levels, use of essential oils has physiological and psychological effects on our physical and emotional well-being. Below is a list of several therapeutic essential oils that are known to be helpful in dealing with mental and emotional problems:

Lavender

Lavender oil is the most commonly used oil for relieving stress and anxiety. Lavender plant contains linalyl and linalool that can pass through the blood brain barrier and affect brain activity almost immediately. According to a recent research that was conducted in 2012, inhaling lavender oil, not only makes one feel relaxed but also makes you feel sharper.

Bergamot

Bergamot is known to stimulate the endocrine system and assists in the production of a sense of calmness and well-being, thus assists in the alleviating of stress levels. Add around 6 drops of bergamot oil to your bathtub and soak in the tub for relief. You can also put five drops of bergamot oil in steaming water in a bowl then place a towel over your head and the bowl to get the steam then inhale for several minutes.

Frankincense

Frankincense has a warm exotic aroma that makes you get the feeling of calmness and relaxation. Inhale this essential oil every time you feel that things are getting out of control; it will do a pretty good job of calming you.

Ylang Ylang

This essential oil is useful in clarifying your thoughts and makes you feel a sense of wellness and calmness. Simply inhaling ylang ylang, will make you feel much better.

Vanilla

The pure scent of vanilla makes you feel at home. Many aroma therapists attribute this to vanilla having the closest scent and flavor to a mother's milk. Vanilla is useful in making you feel relaxed and stimulates mental clarity. Use vanilla in a diffuser and enjoy its amazing scent.

Tangerine

Tangerine is quite effective in enabling you overcome depression.

Lemon

Lemon is essential as it gives a calming, reassuring, and invigorating feeling when inhaled.

Chamomile

Chamomile is also quite effective as a sedative and relaxation aid.

Essential Oils For Pain Relief And Reducing Muscle Spasms

Essential oils for pain relief are effective, as they do not have side effects. I actually believe that essential oils are much better as compared to "over the counter" painkillers like aspirin. There are quite a number of essential oils that have analgesic (means that a substance can reduce or relieve pain) properties.

Birch

This rare essential oil, distilled from the wood of the tree, is very useful when it comes to relieving pain and muscle spasms. Birch essential oil has analgesic (pain reliving), antispasmodic, anti-rheumatic and anti-inflammatory properties that give it the needed edge in fighting pain. It also has methyl salicylate, which acts as 'nature's aspirin'. Birch essential oil is useful in treating:

Arthritis – If you suffer from arthritis, you can relieve pain by applying 1-2 drops of Birch essential oil onto the affected areas. Gently massage the area using a circular motion to relive pain.

Cartilage injury - Massage two drops of the oil into the affected area. Do this at least twice a day.

Cramps – Menstrual cramps can be debilitating for some women. To get relief, massage two drops onto the abdominal area.

Joint pain – In order to alleviate joint pain, use 2-3 drops of the oil, and massage it into the affected joint.

Muscle pain – Muscle pain will ease up if you massage two drops of Birch essential oil into the affected area.

Osteoporosis – Osteoporosis usually comes with age and it's accompanied with pain. To find relief, massage 1-2 drops of the oil onto the painful areas.

Whiplash – When you suffer from whiplash, relieve pain by massaging 1-2 drops of the oil at least twice a day.

After applying Birch essential oil onto an area, you can also use a hot or cold compress on the area depending on the nature of the injury. For example, you can use a hot compress for cramps and a cold compress for muscle pain.

Wintergreen Essential Oil

This is one of my most favorite essential oils when it comes to pain management. Wintergreen has analgesic, anti-inflammatory, and anti-spasmodic properties. It also contains methyl salicylate, which is usually the main ingredient in aspirin; actually, wintergreen contains around 85-99% of methyl salicylate. It is quite interesting to note that wintergreen is among the few plants that contain methyl salicylate naturally. Wintergreen is quite effective against muscle pain, stiff joints, menstrual cramps, ovarian pain, arthritis, and headaches. It can be used for whatever you would use aspirin for. When treating headaches, it is best to inhale wintergreen.

In order to relieve muscle pain, apply wintergreen on the skin. This essential oil also serves as a counterirritant. Counterirritants usually cause irritation that reduces swelling and pain in the underlying tissue. When applying wintergreen essential oil, you should ensure that you dilute it with carrier oil like coconut as it can irritate the skin if not diluted. The percentage of dilution will depend on the listed instructions.

Peppermint Essential Oil

Peppermint is the other essential oil that you can use to manage pain. Peppermint is quite effective since it blocks the channels that transmit pain. It also has anti-inflammatory, antispasmodic, and analgesic properties; hence, it will not only reduce pain and inflammation but also calm spasms that are responsible for causing muscle cramps. Thus, peppermint is one of the most useful essential oils in managing of pain.

Peppermint is quite intense and far more concentrated when compared to other essential oils. Therefore, it is critical to mix with carrier oil like almond oil before applying. It may also not be safe for use on young children.

Lavender

This essential oil is loved by many essential oil enthusiasts including myself for use in relaxation and relief of pain. It is also quite gentle on the skin and is one of the few essential oils that can be used on the skin without diluting. Lavender can be used to treat muscle strain, cramps, and headaches. Additionally, getting a Lavender oil message is effective in easing away back pain as well as tension. You may also inhale lavender oil to treat pain.

Spruce

I especially love spruce essential oil mainly because of its sweet and refreshing scent. Spruce is useful in easing arthritis symptoms as well as lowering back and bone pain. Spruce can be added to massage oils as the aroma is simply amazing and it will soothe muscle pains and pain instantly.

Marjoram

Marjoram can also be referred to as the "happiness herb" mainly because of its sedative properties. It is one of the best essential oils for treating muscle spasms, migraines, stiffness, and arthritis pain. Marjoram is a natural muscle relaxer without all the negative side effects associated with other medications for muscle spasms. Simply dilute the oil using a carrier oil depending on instructions on bottle then rub the essential oil on the affected area.

Sandalwood

Sandalwood essential oil is usually used to treat muscle spasms and back pain. Sandalwood can be inhaled, burned as incense, or applied directly to the skin of course after dilution.

Eucalyptus

This oil has both anti-inflammatory and analgesic properties when used topically. You can use it as a lotion or cream and massage onto the painful areas. It is also useful as a bath salt or oil. Eucalyptus essential oil is effective in treating strains, sprains, nerve pain and muscular aches and pain.

Juniper

Juniper has anti rheumatic and antispasmodic properties that make it the best in reducing muscle spasms, muscle, and joint pains. Juniper is also very helpful in strengthening nerves thus avoiding neuropathic pain.

Chamomile

Chamomile essential oil has anti-inflammatory properties. You can use it to treat muscular and lower back pain as well as severe headaches. You can use chamomile differently to deal with pain. You can steep dried chamomile flowers in hot water and take the tea or you can make the chamomile tea then pour the tea into bath water and enjoy a relaxing bath that will get rid of the pain.

Coriander

Many households around the world use coriander as a spice for flavoring when it comes to cooking meals. However, few households know of its healing properties. Coriander essential oil boasts of its analgesic, anti-rheumatic, anti-inflammatory, antispasmodic and sedative properties. It is useful in treating:

Arthritis – If you suffer from arthritis, you can find relief by massaging two drops of coriander essential oil into the affected area twice a day.

Cartilage injury – Apply 1-2 drops and massage in into the affected area.

Menstrual pain- If experiencing menstrual pain, you can massage 1-2 drops of the oil immediately you start experiencing the symptoms.

Muscles aches – muscle aches can be soothed by massaging 1-2 drops on the affected area. Do this as need arises.

Whiplash – To relieve pain experienced from whiplash, massage 1-2 drops into the area. Do this gently (twice a day) so as not to aggravate the injury.

Another way you can use coriander essential oil is by massaging it into the reflect points of the feet. It would be best if someone can do this for you if you cannot reach all the reflex points.

White Fir

White fir works very well when it comes to relieving pain. This essential oil has anti-arthritic, analgesic, antiseptic, stimulant, anti-catarrhal, and expectorant properties that are useful when dealing with:

Aches: Massage one drop into the aching area (you should dilute the drop with carrier oil before massaging it into your skin)

Cartilage inflammation: Massage one drop into the affected area once daily

Frozen shoulder: Massage two drops on your shoulder when need arises

Muscle fatigue: Massage 1-2 drops working towards the heart area

Muscle pain: Gently massage two drops into the muscle

Rheumatic pain: Massage 1-2 drops on the affected area

Sprain: Massage two drops onto the sprained area

Where pain is concerned, a hot compress will aide in pain relief after you have massaged White Fir on the affected area. However, use a cold compress in case you suffer from a sprain.

Spearmint

Spearmint is a common ingredient in toothpaste and candy. However, it has properties such as anti-inflammatory, anti-spasmodic, anti-catarrhal and stimulant that makes it great for reducing pain and muscle spasms. Spearmint essential oil is extracted when you distill the leaves of the plant. It helps with:

Inflammation: Massage 1-2 drops on the affected area

Headaches: Gently massage two drops onto your forehead area

Muscle spasms and soreness: Massage 1-2 drops on the affected muscles at least twice a day

It is best to dilute the drops with a few drops of carrier oil before applying it to the areas of concern. Rub the spearmint essential oil working towards the heart area, as this will help the lymphatic system as it gets rid of lactic acid.

Essential Oils For Improved Memory And Increased Attention

Mental focus is very important in your ability to undertake day-to-day activities. Unfortunately, at times, circumstances such as accidents and illness cause our mental focus to diminish. Essential oils can improve your memory and boost your mental health.

Clary Sage

Clary sage essential oils has antiseptic, anticonvulsant, antispasmodic, sedative, nerve tonic and warming properties that make it a great ally when it comes to boosting mental health. You should use it for:

Boosting creativity: There are times when your creativity is lacking even as your deadline to hand in a project nears. At times like these, take a drop of clary sage and gently rub it over your brows as you continue to work.

Dealing with depression: If you suffer from depression, massage a drop of clary sage oil on the back of your neck. Also, carry a bottle with you and inhale it throughout the day to improve your mood.

Improving your mood: Mood swings can come unexpectedly; one minute you may feel as if you rule the world and the next, you feel as if the world has fallen and landed on you. When your emotions are all over the place, use clary sage. Breathe it in for a few seconds or rub 1-2 drops onto the soles of your feet.

Dealing with postpartum depression: Giving birth is a wonderful phenomenon that deserves to be celebrated.

Unfortunately, at times it brings about postpartum depression. Use Clary sage to deal with the negative feelings. Rub one or two drops onto your feet and inhale from a bottle several times during the day. Also, diffuse the oil in a room.

Rosemary

Many people use Rosemary in their food or tea not knowing the amazing properties of this essential oil. This essential oil is actually one of the most potent aides as far as mental health is concerned. Rosemary has analgesic, anti-infection, anticancer, anti-inflammatory, antioxidant and expectorant properties. It is useful in:

Clarity: Clarity is needed in order to solve problems, make decisions, and put things into perspective. In order to achieve clarity especially when you are feeling mentally fatigued, cup your hand over your nose and mouth after rubbing a drop of Rosemary oil on it. Inhale for about thirty seconds.

Depression: Depression can quickly color your world and make situations look hopeless. You can uplift your spirits by applying a drop of rosemary essential oil on your hand and cupping your hand over your nose and mouth. Inhale in the oil for up to sixty seconds.

Learning disabilities: If you or a loved one is suffering from a learning disability, use Rosemary to boost your mental power and concentration. Diffuse it in a room or keep a bottle nearby and inhale it several times a day. Also, massage it over your temples and into your toes.

Memory: Rosemary is well known as a memory booster. You should diffuse it in the room or inhale from a bottle from time to time.

Lemongrass

Lemongrass essential oil is useful in revitalizing your mind due to its many healing properties. It is an analgesic, revitalizes, sedative, vasodilator, and antiseptic. Use it for:

Clarity: In order to achieve clarity, rub a drop of Lemongrass essential oil on your hand and use your hand to cover your nose and mouth. Proceed to inhale it in for about half a minute.

Limiting beliefs: Limiting beliefs can prevent you from accomplishing your dreams. When such feelings start cropping up, rub a drop of Lemongrass oil on your hand and cup your hand over your nose and mouth. Inhale for a minimum of thirty seconds.

Mental fatigue: When you are mentally fatigued, you begin to lose your clarity. Use Lemongrass to get it back. Diffuse the essential oil or inhale it from a bottle when the need arises throughout the day.

Peppermint

Many people think of candy or even toothpaste when they hear the word peppermint. However, peppermint essential oil is a powerful healing agent. It is analgesic, antibacterial, antiseptic, antispasmodic, and invigorating. It is useful in:

Alertness: Peppermint essential oil keeps you alert. It is thus a good bet if you are usually sluggish in the morning or during mid-day. Diffuse it into the room or inhale it from the bottle to sharpen your senses.

Memory: When you are under pressure, the stress messes up with your memory, leaving you more frustrated. Peppermint essential oil works to stimulate your mental power and increase your mental process. As you work or study, diffuse the oil into the room you are working from.

Clove

Clove essential oil is extracted from the buds and stem of the plant and it is spicy in nature. It has analgesic, anti-infection, antiseptic, disinfectant, and stimulant properties that enable it to heal the body and mind. Use it for:

Memory: Clove essential oil acts as a memory stimulant. It is thus best to use it when you are studying or working on something. Diffuse the oil and let it work for you as you concentrate on your work. You can also use it topically by diluting it with carrier oil.

Empowerment: Empowerment starts from within your mind. Once you believe you are worth it and that you deserve better, you will start to demand better. Clove essential oil boosts your positivity and helps you accept yourself. You should carry a bottle with you and inhale from it as needed. You can also diffuse the oil in a room.

Control issues: Many theories have been brought forth to explain why some people have control issues. However, the one thing everyone can agree on is that someone who has control issues is unattractive and unpleasant to be around. Use clove essential oil to put you mind at ease. Rub the oil into your feet and diffuse it in a room.

Frankincense

Frankincense essential oil is one of the best-known oils around the world due to its various mentions in various religious books and practices. Frankincense has properties such as antidepressant, stimulant, antitumor, antiseptic, sedative and anticancer that makes it vital when it comes to mental health. Use if for:

Alzheimer's disease: Alzheimer's disease can be devastating both to the sufferer and to his or her family and friends. Fortunately, Frankincense essential oil can help alleviate the symptoms. Use it topically via a body massage or rub it into your feet and soles. Put a drop of the oil on your pillow as you go to sleep at night. Additionally, diffuse the oil in a room during the day.

Brain injury or aging: If you are suffering from the effects of aging or from a brain injury, you can use Frankincense essential oil both topically and aromatically to alleviate your symptoms. Diffuse it as needed and rub into your feet and body. You can also add some drops into your bathing water and soak in it for a while.

Depression: Depression messes up with your mind and thoughts and makes you dwell on negative thoughts. Use Frankincense essential oil and add it into hot steaming water. Use a towel to cover your head, and enclose the steam and inhale the steam.

Prayer and meditation: Frankincense essential oil has been used for centuries during prayer and meditation and for good reason. Frankincense helps you focus and look inwards. It opens up your senses and gives you the clarity you need to answer deep questions. You should diffuse the oil in the room you are using for prayer or meditation. You can also apply it on your hands, on your feet and on your forehead during this time.

Memory: Frankincense essential oil is a great study aide as it sharpens your mind and enables you to retain and recall what you have studied or what you are working on. Add two drops of the oil in hot water in a bowl, cover your head with towel over bowl, and inhale until the steam stops. Ensure that you use a towel to cover your head and trap the steam. You can also massage the oil into your toes and soles.

Mental fatigue: When you are suffering from mental fatigue, there is not much you can do in terms of activities especially the ones that require you to solve problems. However, you can get relief by massaging Frankincense into your scalp. You can also rub it across your chest and use it in your bath water to settle your mind.

Your mental health is important and should not be ignored especially when you can use essential oils to ensure that your mind stays healthy and sharp. Identify which essential oils work best for you, and use them to improve your mental health.

Essential Oils For Treating Skin Infections

As the biggest organ in your body, your skin should be well protected from harmful pathogens and harsh weather. Fungi, bacteria, viruses, dirt, and disease all work to cause your skin harm. However, you can use essential oils to care for your skin and treat infections.

Bergamot

The healing effects of Bergamot essential oil have already been discussed. Bergamot also has antibacterial, antiparasitic, antiseptic, and anti-infectious properties that make it useful in healing your skin. You can use it for:

Acne: Use Bergamot to cure acne by dabbing it over the blemish. Once you have applied it to your skin, stay away from direct sunlight to avoid sensitization.

Cold sores: Apply Bergamot essential oil as soon as you notice a cold sore forming. Use a drop directly on the sore. You can also dilute the drop with coconut oil. Apply the mixture at least three times a day.

Eczema: Eczema is a skin condition that can be treated by using a drop of Bergamot essential oil mixed with a teaspoon of coconut oil. Ensure that you gently massage the oil into the area at least twice a day.

Oily skin: Oily skin attracts dirt and germs. As your pores clog, the situation escalates to pimples and acne. If you have oily skin, use Bergamot essential oil. Its astringent property will work to improve the condition of your skin. Apply one drop topically each day. Ensure that you first do a skin patch test before massaging the oil into your skin. Keep away from sunlight once you have applied the oil.

Varicose veins: Varicose veins are not pretty by any standards. Apply a drop of Bergamot essential oil on the area and massage very gently at least twice a day.

Chamomile

Chamomile is often mentioned when it comes to skin care products. Its properties such as anti-inflammatory, anti-infectious, anti-parasitic, and relaxing make it useful in dealing with:

Bruises: Gently massage a drop of the oil over the bruise. Ensure that you do not massage the area vigorously as this could bring about blood clots.

Cuts: Chamomile is used to reduce inflammation and promote the healing of cuts and scrapes. Massage a drop over the area or use a hot compress over the area.

Rashes: In order to soothe irritated skin, use a drop of chamomile and mix it with three drops of carrier oil before massaging it into the affected area.

Dermatitis: Add chamomile essential oil to your lotion and use it daily.

Juniper berry

Juniper berry essential oil is a useful oil when it comes to skin care. It has antiseptic, astringent, tonic, diuretic, and detoxifier properties. It is useful when it comes to dealing with acne for instance. Simply wash your face before applying one to two drops of the oil after dilution. If you have other skin problems, add one to two drops of the oil to your moisturizer or mix it with coconut oil and make it part of your daily skin care routine.

Patchouli

Many people are divided when it comes to loving or hating Patchouli but what they can agree on is that it has awesome properties that are very useful when it comes to skin care. It has anti-inflammatory, antifungal, antiseptic, and astringent properties. It is useful when dealing with acne, dandruff, Dermatitis, Hives, Rash, stretch marks etc.

Gently massage one or two drops into the affected area. Patchouli can be applied directly but you can dilute it with a moisturizing carrier whenever you want to use it especially if you have sensitive skin.

Thyme

Thyme essential oil is useful when dealing with various skin ailments. It is derived from the flowers, leaves, and stem, and has antifungal, antibacterial, antioxidant, antiviral, and antiseptic properties that make it useful when dealing with insect bites, stings, dermatitis, eczema, and fungal infections.

It is best to dilute a drop of the oil with carrier oil such as coconut oil before applying it to an affected area. Use the oil at least twice a day.

Many essential oils can be used as part of your skin care routine. Find out which one works for you and ensure you use the essential oils wisely to prevent further inflammation in case your skin is sensitive to the oil. Perform a skin patch test to be sure of the oil.

Essential Oils For Overcoming Addictions

When you have an addiction, your life will pretty much revolve around satisfying that addiction. The thing with addictions is that it is hard to get rid of them. They cause intense cravings that just have to be satisfied and even when you get rid of an addiction, you go through withdrawal symptoms that can cause you to return to your addiction. Essential oils are good in treating addictions because they work to stop that craving. Without the craving, you will be less tempted to indulge in your addiction especially if you are bent on completely getting rid of an addiction. In order to treat addiction, you can use essential oils such as:

Black pepper

Black pepper is often used as a spice. This essential oil is extracted by steam distilling its berries (the Piperceae berries). It is an antiseptic, analgesic, laxative, stimulant, antispasmodic, antitoxic, and anti-inflammatory amongst other properties. Use black pepper essential oil for:

Curing addictions: One of the addictions a lot of people try to get rid off is tobacco addiction. Tobacco is bad for you. You already know this but you may have tried to quit smoking to no avail. Use black pepper essential oil to stop your cravings. Take a small amount of the oil and place it on your tongue when you crave tobacco. Dilute it with carrier oil (edible) if it is too strong. Also, diffuse the oil during the day to keep cravings away.

Emotional support: When you are trying to quit something you are addicted to, you will need all the emotional support you can get. Black pepper essential oil provides this support.

Dilute one drop of the oil with a carrier oil and proceed to massage it on your heart center. You can also diffuse the oil.

Journaling: One of the major things people with addictions have to battle is the lies they tell themselves. You may have an addiction but you may continue telling yourself 'it is not that serious' or 'I can stop whenever I want to'. Black pepper essential oil gets rids of superficiality and allows you to be truthful to yourself as you put your thoughts down on paper.

Basil

Over the years, Basil has been known as the oil of renewal due to its energizing and restorative properties. Basil essential oil can be also used to overcome addictions. Basil essential oil has anti-infectious, antioxidant, antidepressant, anti-inflammatory, antispasmodic, antiviral, decongestant, diuretic, uplifting and stimulant properties that help with mental healing. Use Basil for:

Addiction: Addiction can be hard to overcome if you don't have a way to deal with the cravings that often spring up. Use Basil essential oil to deal with cravings. You can diffuse the oil in a room. You can also massage it over your heart and solar plexus. In addition, you can carry a bottle with you to inhale when you have cravings.

Nervousness: Many people get nervous especially when they have to do something in front of an audience. Many use alcohol or tobacco to get over their nerves. However, this often leads to addiction. In order to calm your nerves, use Basil essential oil. You can inhale the oil straight from the bottle, or you can first rub a drop on your hand and hold it over your nose and mouth for half a minute.

Grapefruit

Many people enjoy eating grapefruits but they give no thought to what happens to its rind after they dispose it. The rind is the one that is cold compressed to extract grapefruit essential oil. Grapefruit essential oil has antidepressant, diuretic, stimulant, disinfectant and antiseptic properties. Use it for:

Addiction: Stop drug cravings by inhaling the aroma of Grapefruit essential oil straight from the bottle. You can also massage one drop of the oil over your stomach or over the back of your neck.

Food addiction: Food addiction often leads to eating disorders and obesity. In order to cure addiction to food, add one to two drops of Grapefruit essential oil to your drinking water.

Sugar cravings: When you have a 'sweet tooth', you tend to crave sugar even when you know you've already had too much. However, you can stop the cravings by using Grapefruit essential oil. When the craving strikes, inhale the oil from the bottle for a few seconds. You can also add a drop to your drinking water and take this at least twice a day.

Withdrawal: One of the major things that stop people from successfully quitting their addictions is the withdrawal symptoms. Fortunately, Grapefruit essential oil not only curbs your cravings but it also alleviates withdrawal symptoms. Diffuse the oil in a room and you can also massage a drop of the oil over your throat and back of the neck.

Bergamot

Bergamot essential oil is rich in establishing emotional wellness. It has uplifting, anti-infections, neuroprotective, sedative, antispasmodic and antiseptic properties that are useful for mental health. You should use it for:

Addictions: In order to curb addictions, you should massage a drop of Bergamot essential oil over you solar plexus. You should also proceed to massage one drop into your feet. Do this twice a day and ensure that you diffuse the oil in a room.

Compulsions: Compulsions can drive you mad especially when you are trying to stop yourself from acting on them. Use Bergamot essential oil to help you in your struggle. Massage a drop of the oil into your feet and another drop over your solar plexus. Do this at least twice a day.

Confidence: Many people turn to addictive products in the hopes of gaining confidence. However, this is a false confidence that wears off once the effects of the product diminishes but it leaves the individual craving more of the product. Use Bergamot essential oil to boost your confidence levels. Rub a drop of the oil into your hand and hold your hand over your nose and mouth then inhale for at least one minute. You can also massage the oil over your abdomen as needed.

Depression: Depression affects your life simply because it colors your world in dark colors. You can use Bergamot essential oil to improve your mood instead of turning to harmful substances. Rub a drop into your hand before holding your hand over your nose and mouth. Take a few seconds just to inhale it.

Stress: Stress is one of the leading factors blamed for addiction. And when you are addicted to something, stress only makes you crave it more. When you are feeling stressed, inhale Bergamot essential oil directly from the bottle. You can also massage a drop into your hands, feet, or abdomen when you need to.

Limiting beliefs: When you have limiting beliefs, you may find yourself turning to addictive substances in an attempt to boost your confidence. Instead of turning to substances that will eventually only harm you, use Bergamot essential oil to change your beliefs. Inhale from the bottle whenever you are feeling down. Also, massage one drop of the oil into your feet and hands.

Clove

Clove essential oil is extracted from the plant's bud and stem. It has analgesic, anti-infectious, antiseptic, antioxidant, antitumor, disinfectant and stimulant properties that make it great for healing. Clove is used for promoting healthy emotional boundaries. Use it for:

Addiction: In order to cure addiction, use Clove essential oil. When the craving strikes, apply a drop of the oil to the tip of your tongue. If you find it too strong, dilute the drop with carrier oil like coconut oil before using it.

Boundaries: Boundaries are a necessary part of life. When you don't have boundaries, people tend to take advantage of you. But sometimes, you may find it hard to set boundaries and turn to alcohol or drugs in an effort to fit in. Diffuse clove essential oil or massage in over your heart and solar plexus to get your life back on track.

Codependency: When you are dependent on something in order to function, your life starts revolving around that something. Use Clove essential oil to do away with dependency. Inhale the essential oil straight from the bottle.

Diffuse it when you are writing down your thoughts or when you are meditating. This will foster your will and make you stand on your own.

Yes, essential oils will be a great help in curing addictions. However, you also need to bolster your chances of success by adopting a healthy lifestyle. Resist temptation by staying away from the thing you are addicted to and use some mental exercises to bolter your will.

Essential Oils For The Respiratory System

The nose, throat, sinuses and all sacks and tubes of air passage cannot do their work if they are inflamed or clogged. Since the digestive and the respiratory systems are closely related, you would need to watch what you eat as this will affect your respiratory system. Some of the foods that are known to cause a majority of the respiratory problems are dairy products like milk, processed sugars and highly processed grains and starches. If you would want to overcome a respiratory problem, it is advisable that you limit your intake of dairy products, sweeteners and highly processed foods. Below is a list of various respiratory conditions that you may find yourself having, and how best to treat them by use of essential oils.

Sore throat

When you have a sore throat, you can use different essential oils and varied methods to deal with the soreness.

*You can for instance take a trace of frankincense or tea tree and pour it on the back of your hand, lick it and transfer it to the back of your throat. Mix it with saliva and coat the inflamed tissues. Repeat the process every minute or two until you feel some relief, then you can decrease the frequency as the soreness reduces.

*You may also use a few drops of tea tree oil and apply them on the areas on your throat where there are inflamed lymph nodes to the main bone behind your ear to the center of your throat.

Colds and Flu

Colds and Flu are very common especially during winter with the climate change and there being less exposure to sunshine. Although most people turn to antibiotics including myself (a while back) you can use antiviral essential oils to get relief.

*If you want to clear a blocked nose, you can mix peppermint with honey. Then hold the mixture at the back of your throat until the peppermint vapors get to the sinuses to open up the air passage.

*You can also apply eucalyptus on your throat and the bone behind your ear.

*You can also use other essential oils like oregano, cinnamon, basil, and lemon to treat colds and flu.

Sinusitis

In most cases, inflammation of the sinuses is usually due to upper respiratory infection. When suffering from sinusitis, you are likely to have different symptoms including loss of the ability to smell, a blocked nose, severe headache, facial pain and mucous discharge. Some essential oils can treat both the sinusitis as well as its symptoms. For instance, you can rub a few drops of frankincense or peppermint on each temple to ease a sinus headache. If you have a stuffy nose, you can mix a teaspoon of honey with a drop of peppermint and hold it at the back of your mouth until the vapor moves to the back of your throat.

You can also do steam inhalations of lavender, lemon and myrrh. Deep breaths through the nose will ensure that upper respiratory infections do not spread to the sinuses. Steam inhalations are usually effective when you have an upper respiratory infection as they prevent the spread of the infection into the sinuses.

Asthma

Asthma is usually triggered by the presence of fungus, pollen, and dust in the air. The use of essential oils has been known to relax and open the air passage thus fight infections safely. When using essential oils, it is advisable not to inhale them, as the lungs are very sensitive to any allergic trigger. You may actually make the condition worse by inhaling the oils.

To make breathing much easier, you should apply 2 drops of fir or aspire or eucalyptus radiata to the toes, upper back, upper chest and nape of the neck. Use these essential oils on a daily basis to fight infections.

Pneumonia

Pneumonia refers to a wide array of lung inflammations; some are viral while some are bacterial. The common symptoms are usually the production of mucous, sweating, high fever, shortness of breath and chest pain. If you have ever suffered from pneumonia, you know that this is a very serious condition since the small air sacks in the lungs are filled with pus and red blood cells making it difficult to get enough oxygen through the lungs. You can, however, use essential oils under the guidance of a professional to enable you enjoy the healing benefits of essential oils.

Diffuse tea tree, eucalyptus, and deliverance to restore vitality to the lungs. It is advisable to alternate between these essential oils to get the maximum benefits from each of them. The use of frankincense and peppermint is important to ward off secondary sinus infections. You can put the essential oil on the tongue; hold it for some time then swallow.

Steam inhalations of fir and lavender are also effective in helping with coughing spasms. You should simmer 2 cups of water and add 3-6 drops of essential oil. Take a towel, place over your head, and inhale the steam vapors. You should do this several times a day to break the mucous and assist in relieving the inflammation.

Bronchitis

A cold can easily lead to the inflammation of the trachea and bronchial tubes. This leads to the frequent coughing spells that are associated with bronchitis. There is a variety of ways that you can use essential oils to treat bronchitis or reduce the symptoms of this condition.

Add a drop of aspire, which is usually a combination of cypress, eucalyptus, marjoram, peppermint, rosemary, spruce and myrtle to your humidifier to purify the air.

Before using any essential oils to treat different respiratory conditions, it is advisable to seek advice from your health professional with adequate knowledge about the use of essential oils to treat different respiratory problems.

Essential Oils For Digestive Disorders

The digestive system includes the mouth, esophagus, small intestine, large intestine, stomach, rectum, and anus. Digestive disorders range from simple stomach upsets to severe ones like having colon cancers. Different types of essential oils can be used for varied digestive disorders.

Peppermint

In addition to peppermint creating a calming effect on the body when inhaled, it also allows the release of painful gas from the stomach as well as reducing intestinal spasms. Peppermint can also offer relief when you experience menstrual cramps and diarrhea or suffer from irritable bowel syndrome. Owing to the antiviral, antibacterial and antifungal properties of peppermint, it is also useful in fighting any harmful organisms present in the digestive system.

Lavender

As indicated above, lavender is useful in calming the nervous system and this helps relieve various digestive disorders.

Tarragon Oil

This essential oil has a wide array of uses including stimulation of digestive function. Tarragon has also been used to fight intestinal worms. It is also useful in the stimulation of the natural production of bile that is essential in the assimilation of fats and other nutrients by the body in addition to elimination of toxins from the body.

Lemon essential oil

Ingestion of this oil is beneficial as it stimulates the liver as well as detoxifies the body. You can also apply lemon topically although when you do so, you should remember that lemon is phototoxic; hence, you should not apply on the skin before going out in the sun.

Clove Essential Oil

Taking clove oil can assist in the alleviating of symptoms associated with the inflammation of the intestinal lining that can cause digestive comfort. Clove oil is quite effective as it relaxes the muscle lining of the digestive tract and helps prevent nausea, bloating, diarrhea, gas, and intestinal spasms. If you have yeast infections or fungal overgrowths that can interfere with digestion, taking clove oil can be a sure way of treating these fungal infections. Taking clove oil with meals is also helpful as the oil stimulates digestive function in addition to energizing the body.

Cardamom oil

This essential oil is one of my favorite oils as it stimulates digestion thus maintaining a well-functioning digestive tract. Cardamom is essential in treating common disorders like constipation, diverticulitis, and acid reflux disease mainly due to its ability to stimulate the balanced secretion of gastric juices and bile.

Lemongrass essential oil

This is one of the best essential oils owing to it being a digestive tonic. It is also very useful in calming nausea.

Fennel Essential Oil

Fennel is the best known for use when dieting as it is effective in detoxifying. You can take fennel internally as an herbal tea and not in the form of an essential oil.

Cinnamon

This powerful antimicrobial essential oil is useful in treating an aching belly and fighting infection. It is also very useful in boosting the metabolism. However, when using cinnamon, you need to use it sparingly because it can be quite irritating to the skin.

Ginger essential oil

The essential oil from this root is beneficial in toning the digestive system. Ginger is most suitable if you experience nausea and are vomiting.

Essential Oils For Improved Immune System
And Repair Of Damaged Tissue

In order for your damaged tissue to be of use again, there is need for adequate healing and repair. Scarring after a wound, skin inflammation or injury is usually a very critical part of the healing process that may take some time depending on the damage to the tissue. However, several essential oils have been known to have the ability to support both the immune system and improve one's healing rate. Some of these oils improve the immune system by stimulating the production of white blood cells while others encourage new cell growth thus promoting faster healing. It is usually best to improve your immune system by having a lymphatic massage with the use of essential oils. Lymph nodes located throughout the body are like filtering centers for cleaning the blood and the lymphatic system usually moves cellular fluid through the entire system cleansing the body of any waste thus the use of essential oils is quite good at stimulating movement thus supporting the cleansing process.

Some essentials that are suitable for improving the immune system and regenerating damaged tissue include:

Lemongrass Essential oil

You can use lemongrass for treating tendons, ligaments, cartilage, and regenerating connective tissue. You can also use it for repairing muscles, bones, and ligaments.

Helichrysum

This is the oil of choice if you are looking to heal scar tissue both old and recent. It usually stops bleeding by coagulation and assists in the repair of the tissue. You can also add carrier oil and apply it directly to your acne, stretch markets, wounds, and surgical scars. Its ability to cause the regeneration of tissues is due to the presence of diketone, the 3rd major component.

Helichrysum is also useful in nerve damage repair. The use of helichrysum in several cases of deafness in children born deaf has been seen to lead to the regeneration of nerves in the ears; deafness caused by inability of nerves to connect has been cured by the use of helichrysum.

Sandalwood

Sandalwood essential oil is quite useful in scarring. All you need to do is apply sparingly to the respective scar area overnight and over time, the scar will diminish in appearance.

Cypress

This is one of the mostly used essential oils for the lymphatic system. It is anti-bacterial, anti-infectious and is useful in relieving lymphatic problems.

Tea Tree Oil

Tea tree oil is useful in avoiding infection and is useful in preventing scarring. It is important to note that this oil does not remove existing scars.

Garlic Oil

This is the most suitable essential oil if you are susceptible to continued infection. You should use garlic oil on the feet after diluting it 4% with your favorite carrier oil like coconut oil, olive oil or jojoba oil.

You can use these essential oils differently depending on your skin's sensitivity to the oil and the effectiveness of the oil. For instance, you can use aromatherapy by inhaling the essential oil, ingesting it, or applying it topically on your skin. You can also consider infusing a suitable immunity-building essential oil into the air that you breathe. The most suitable way of achieving this is by use of an ultrasonic aromatherapy diffuser, which are the best in maintaining the integrity of the essential oil for therapeutic use. They are also effective in purifying the air and distributing negative ions that are helpful in improving flow of oxygen to the brain.

Essential Oils With Anti-Aging Properties

Essential oils play a critical role in anti-aging skin care routine. This is mainly due to the regenerative properties of essential oils. Essential oils usually have proteins and nutrients found in anti-aging oils that encourage cell regeneration and maintain the elasticity and firmness of the skin. Some of these important essential oils include:

Rosewood oil

This essential oil is very effective in improving your skin's elasticity and firmness while reducing the appearance of deep wrinkles, brown age spots, and fine lines. Rosewood also diminishes stretch marks, wrinkles and scars thus ensuring that your skin is tight, firm, young and most of all healthy.

Clary sage

Clary sage contains antioxidants that are useful in reversing the signs of aging like skin discoloration and wrinkles. This is usually possible due to the antioxidants protecting your skin against free radicals that are damaging to the skin causing aging. This essential oil also has antibacterial and antiseptic properties that assist in the tightening of pores, making the skin firm and tight.

Myrrh Oil

This oil has a great reputation when it comes to essential oils in aromatherapy. It is also suitable in rejuvenating aging skin mainly due to its anti-inflammatory and antiseptic properties. This natural oil is also known to improve dull and dry skin on your face and neck in addition to treating blemishes pigmentation and sun damaged skin.

Patchouli

This oil is made from leaves of the patchouli bush. Its anti-aging properties make it suitable for use on all skin types. In most cases, you are likely to find many wrinkle creams having patchouli oil as their main ingredient. Owing to the anti-inflammatory properties of patchouli essential oil, it is perfect for use on mature skin that is usually prone to acne. It also reduces pores, removes wrinkles and fine lines while tightening sagging skin.

Frankincense Essential oil

Frankincense is best for reducing wrinkles, removing scars and stretch marks. It is also useful in restoring elasticity to the skin especially around the eyes.

Lavender Essential oil

This is one of the most versatile oils owing to its many uses. Lavender is useful as an anti-aging essential oil since it is a skin regenerator thus lightening the appearance of age spots and reducing scaring from wounds.

Bonus Chapter: Essential Oil Recipes

As a special and time limited bonus, I included the 33 top essential oil recipes from my other book as well.

Essential Oil Recipe for Arthritis

Ingredients

- 2 ounces of carrier oil (jojoba, pomegranate seed oil)

- 20 drops of Roman Chamomile

- 5 drops of black pepper

Blend all the oils together and store in an airtight glass container -preferably a dark-colored glass container. You may also substitute the black pepper with 10 drops of Helichrysum and reduce the amount of Roman Chamomile to 10 drops while maintaining the same amount of carrier oil.

Use a small amount of the oil blend to massage gently into arthritic joints. In order to know how best to massage your joints, you may need to speak to your doctor. In case of any discomfort, you can discontinue use.

Arthritic Joint Soaking Bath Essential Oil Recipe

Ingredients

- 4 drops of juniper berry

- 2 drops of cypress

- 2 drops of Rosemary

- 2 drops of Lavender

- 1 cup of Bath salt Blend

Instructions

Add this blend to a bath just after filling or while filing and soak for twenty to thirty minutes.

Essential Oil Recipe for Menstrual cramps

Ingredients

- 1 ounce of jojoba

- 3 drops of Lavender Essential oil

- 4 drops of Peppermint Essential Oil

- 4 drops of Cypress Essential oil

Instructions

Mix the oils in a clean, dark-colored glass bottle. Each time you experience cramps, gently massage a small amount of the oil blend in the abdominal area.

Stress Relief Essential oil blend

Ingredients

- 2 drops of petitgrain

- 1 drop of ylang ylan

- 2 drops of Lavender

- 5 tsp of carrier oil (coconut, jojoba)

Instructions

Mix all the oils thoroughly in a dark-colored glass bottle. Use the oil blend to mix and massage onto the body.

Insomnia Essential Oil Blend

Ingredients

- 1 drop of clary sage

- 3 drops of Lavender

- 1 tsp of cream or milk

Instructions

Mix the ingredients until well blended. Add the oil blend to a warm bath and soak.

Essential oil Blend for congestion

Ingredients

- 4 drops of Peppermint Essential oil

- 26 drops of Ravensara Essential oil

- 30 drops of Eucalyptus Essential oil

Cotton Ball

Instructions

Blend the essential oils in a dark colored glass bottle (clean), preferably with a built-in dropper. Apply two or three drops of the essential oil blend to the cotton ball and inhale occasionally until your nose clears.

Intestinal Ailments Essential Oil Blend

Ingredients

- 1 drop of clove oil

- 2 drops of Rosemary oil

- 1 drop of peppermint oil

- 1 drop of chamomile oil

- 5 ml vegetable carrier oil

Instructions

Blend the essential oils thoroughly. Rub the essential oil blend on the belly or the area of discomfort.

Acne Essential oil Blend

Ingredients

- 1 ounce of jojoba

- 1 drop of Geranium Essential oil

- 6 drops of Lavender Essential oil

- 5 drops of Tea Tree essential oil

Instructions

Pour the jojoba oil in a clean bottle then add the essential oils and close the bottle. Roll the bottle gently for two minutes to mix the oils. Apply a small amount of the oil blend to the neck, back and face while avoiding lips, nostrils and eyes. Apply to affected areas twice every day to freshly cleansed skin. Ensure that you role the bottle gently each time before use to make sure that the oils are thoroughly mixed.

Essential oil Recipe for Stress Relief

Ingredients

- 1 drop of chamomile essential oil or ylang ylang

- 1 drop of Rose Geranium Essential oil

- 4 drops of Lavender essential oil

- 4 drops of Orange Essential oil

- 10 drops of Bergamot essential oil

- 1 tsp of coarse sea salt

Instructions

Pour the coarse sea salt in a very small dark glass bottle then add the essential oils. For stress relief, take three long, slow and deep breaths of the essential blend, take a short break and take more deep breathes. Do this around three times to get the required stress relief.

Essential oil Blend for Bruises

Ingredients

- 8 drops of Helichrysum Essential oil

- 1 ounce of Sweet almond oil and jojoba

Instructions

Mix the Helichrysum essential oil and the jojoba or sweet almond oil and store in a dark colored bottle. Apply the oil blend lightly on bruises one or two times a day.

Essential oil Balm for Minor scrapes and cuts

Ingredients

- 40 drops of Tea Tree Oil

- 40 drops of lavender Oil

- 3 ounces of vegetable carrier oil like sweet almond oil or jojoba oil

- 1 ounce of grated beeswax

Instructions

Place the beeswax in a double boiler and melt the wax on low heat. Slowly and gently, heat your jojoba or sweet almond oil in a pan over low heat. Pour the warm carrier oil into a bowl and add the melted beeswax then stir well.

Add in the tea tree and lavender essential oils and stir again then pour the mixture in a wide mouth jar. Allow it to cool for a few minutes before you put the lid on.

Wait for some time until the ointment has cooled before using it.

Once you have cleaned the cut, apply a small amount of the balm and apply a bandage if need be.

High blood pressure essential oil Blend

Ingredients

- 1 ounce of carrier oil

- 10 drops of ylang ylang essential oil

- 5 drops of cypress essential oil

- 5 drops of marjoram essential oil

Instructions

Simply blend the oils together and rub the mixture over your heart and on the heart reflexology points on the left hand and left foot.

Essential oil recipe for Ringworm and Athlete's Foot

Ingredients

- 2 drops of tea tree essential oil

- 1 tsp of carrier oil

- 1 drop of lavender essential oil

Instructions

Mix the oils together thoroughly and store in a dark colored glass bottle. Apply on the specific area using a cotton swab.

Essential oil Recipe for Flu, colds and coughs

Ingredients

- 2 drops of eucalyptus essential oil

- 2 drops of lavender essential oil

- 2 drops of tea tree essential oil

Instructions

Boil a pot of water and remove from the heat source. While steaming, add in the eucalyptus, lavender and tea tree essential oils. Cover your head with a towel as you inhale the steam for at least three minutes. Always ensure that your eyes are closed.

Recipe For easing coughs

Ingredients

- 2 drops of lavender essential oil

- 2 drops of eucalyptus essential oil

Instructions

Boil a pot of water and remove from the heat. As it is still steaming, add the eucalyptus and lavender oils. Immediately, cover the pot and your head with a towel and inhale the steam for around three minutes while your eyes are closed. If you would want to ease the coughing throughout the day, it is advisable to add the eucalyptus oil and lavender to a carrier oil and apply on your chest and throat.

Essential oil blend for Muscle pain and Aches

Ingredients

- 2 drops of rosemary essential oil

- 2 drops of lavender essential oil

- 4 tsp of carrier oil

Instructions

Mix the oils and use to massage the area with the muscle pain.

When having a headache, massage two drops of Lavender essential oil on your temple.

Anti wrinkle Essential oil Blend

Ingredients

- 10 drops of frankincense essential oil

- 10 drops of neroli essential oil

- 10 drops of lavender essential oil

- 10 drops of Fennel Essential oil

- 3 drops of Lemon essential oil

- 10 drops of carrot seed essential oil

- 10 drops of Evening Primrose oil

- 2 tbsp of one of these oils- sweet almond, hazelnut or Apricot Kernel

- 2 drops of Rosemary essential oil

Instructions

Blend all the ingredients in a bottle. Once well blended, apply a few drops of the essential oil blend to the neck and face each night right after toning your skin.

Hair Loss Essential oil Blend

Ingredients

- 1 tbsp of sweet almond oil

- 1 tbsp of jojoba oil

- 4 drops of Rosemary essential oil

- 6 drops of clary sage essential oil

- 4 drops of Roman chamomile essential oil

- 10 drops of lavender essential oil

- 40 drops of carrot seed essential oil

Instructions

Blend all the oils in a clean bottle. Shake well before use. It is usually advisable to warm the oils then apply a few drops on the scalp until it is absorbed in or overnight. Apply a couple of times each week.

Essential oil blend for treating scabies and lice

Ingredients

- 5 ml of carrier oil

- 1 drop of thyme essential oil

- 2 drops of cinnamon essential oil

- 2 drops of rosemary essential oil

- 2 drops of pine essential oil

Instructions

Mix the oils and apply them directly on the affected area. Before use, ensure you perform a skin test on the inside part of the forearm.

Essential oils Blend to Soften calluses and corns

Ingredients

- 2 tbsp of sunflower or sweet almond oils

- 2 drops of Roman chamomile

- 20 drops of tagetes

- 5 drops of carrot seed essential oil

Instructions

Mix these oils in a bottle and apply a few drops on the corn two times daily. You may continue using this blend periodically when you have a corn or as a way of preventing the calluses and/or corns from returning.

Varicose veins massage oil blend

Ingredients

- 4 drops of cypress oil

- 2 drops of Wheat germ oil

- 4 drops of lavender oil

- 20 ml of almond oil

Instructions

Mix the oils and massage on your legs gently every day

Toothache massage oil

Ingredients

- 1 drop of lemon oil

- 1 drop of clove oil

- 3 drops of chamomile oil

- 5 ml of vegetables oil

Instructions

Mix these oils, massage on the cheek, and jawbone to ease the pain.

Massage oil to reduce fever

Ingredients

- 1 drop of tea tree essential oil

- 1 drop of rosemary essential oil

- 2 drops of peppermint essential oil

- 1 drop of black pepper essential oil

- 2 drops eucalyptus essential oil

- 2 drops of lavender essential oil

- 15 ml of evening primrose oil

Instructions

Mix the oils and massage your temples, soles of feet, tops of hands and the back of your neck.

Heartburn essential oil blend

Ingredients

- 1 drop of peppermint essential oil

- 2 drops of eucalyptus essential oil

- 2 drops of fennel oil

- 1 tsp of grape seed oil

Mix these oils and use the blend to rub the upper abdominal area.

Essential oil mouthwash for fighting gingivitis

Ingredients

- 1 tbsp of brandy

- 3 drops of peppermint essential oil

- 3 drops of thyme essential oil

- 3 drops of chamomile essential oil

- 2 drops of eucalyptus essential oil

Instructions

Mix the oils and dissolve one tsp of the mixture in a glass of warm water. Swish the warm water and oil mixture in your mouth but do not swallow.

Essential oil mouthwash for ulcers

Ingredients

- 2 drops of tea tree oil

- 2 drops of geranium oil

- 2 drops of thyme oil

- 2 drops of lemon oil

- 2 drops of peppermint oil

- 10 ml brandy

Instructions

Mix all the oils and dissolve a teaspoon in a glass of water, swish around your mouth then spit out.

Essential oil mouthwash to help with bleeding gums

Ingredients

- 3 drops of peppermint oil

- 3 drops of thyme

- 3 drops of chamomile oil

- 2 drops of eucalyptus oil

- 1 tbsp of brandy

Instructions

Mix these oils and dissolve in one tablespoon of brandy. Use a teaspoon of the oils in a glass of warm water. Swish the warm water with the mixture around your mouth, then spit; do not swallow.

Essential oil blend for treating boils

Ingredients

- 2 drops of tea tree oil

- 2 drops of lavender oil

- 1 drop of juniper oil

- 200 ml of water

Instructions

Bathe the infected area with this mixture twice daily. If the inflammation is too severe, you can add a drop of chamomile essential oil.

Chapped lips Essential oil Blend

Ingredients

- 2 drops of rose oil

- 2 drops of geranium oil

- 1 drop of neroli oil

- 20 ml of aloe vera oil

Instructions

Apply this oil mixture on chapped lips, as it is helpful in easing pain and in healing of the lips.

Massage oil blend to help with difficulty in breathing

Ingredients

- 3 drops of rosemary oil

- 10 drops of eucalyptus oil

- 10 drops of ginger oil

- 5 drops of nutmeg oil

- 2 drops of cinnamon oil

- 30 ml of vegetable carrier oil

Instructions

This massage oil mixture needs to be rubbed around the back and chest.

Essential oil blend for Anal Fissures

You can consider washing the area with warm water with five drops of lemon oil and lavender oil. You can use a massage oil to deal with the abdominal pain.

Ingredients

- 1 drop of peppermint oil

- 1 drop of chamomile oil

- 1 drop of clove oil

- 5 ml of carrier oil

Instructions

Mix these oils and massage the stomach gently in a clockwise motion.

Essential oil mouthwash to fight bad breath

Ingredients

- 4 drops of lavender oil

- 5ml brandy

- 125 ml of warm water

Mix all these ingredients together and use this mixture when required by swirling around the mouth after brushing your teeth and flossing. Ensure you spit it out. Do not swallow.

Essential oil Blend to ease diarrhea

Ingredients

- 2 drops of eucalyptus oil

- 2 drops of lavender oil

- 2 drops of chamomile oil

- 2 drops of peppermint oil

- 2 drops of geranium oil

- 10 ml of vegetable oil

Instructions

Mix these essential oils and rub over the abdomen area.

Conclusion

Essential oils have a wide array of uses such that I cannot begin to list all of them. These oils are frequently used through inhalation, ingestion and applying topically to the specific areas. As you use essential oils, it is important to know that most of them cannot be used on the skin without diluting. You should also seek medical advice from your healthcare provider before using different essential oils. For instance, if you are pregnant, you cannot use some essential oils. If you suffer from hypertension, you should be cautious about the use of essential oils. The use of essential oils is quite beneficial especially since they treat different ailments without the harmful side effects associated with drugs.

I really hope that you liked this book and that I could help you to get started with essential oils and aromatherapy. If you liked this book, I'd like to ask you for a favor: Would you be so kind to leave a review on amazon? It'd be VERY much appreciated!

Always to your success,

Sarah

Made in the USA
San Bernardino, CA
25 June 2015